CW00569852

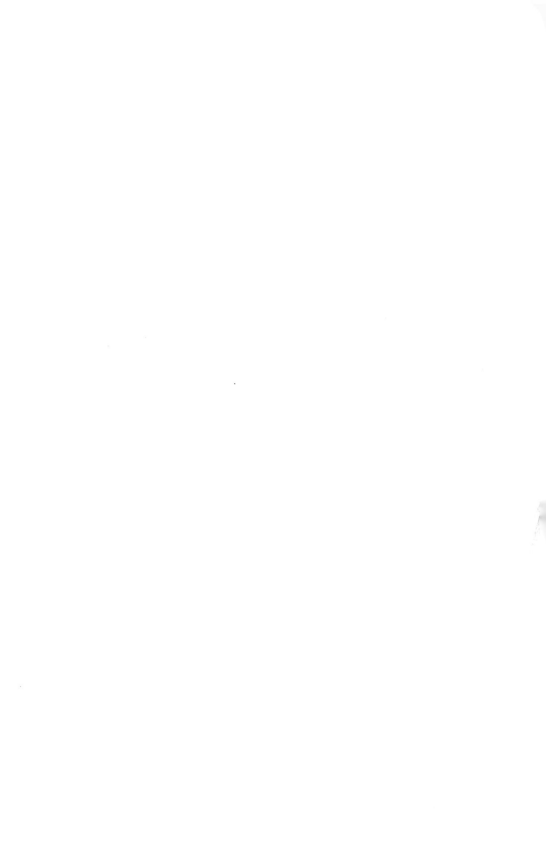

# The Complete Keto Recipes Cookbook

## Quick and Easy Recipes To Boost Your Brain and Improve Your Health

Otis Fisher

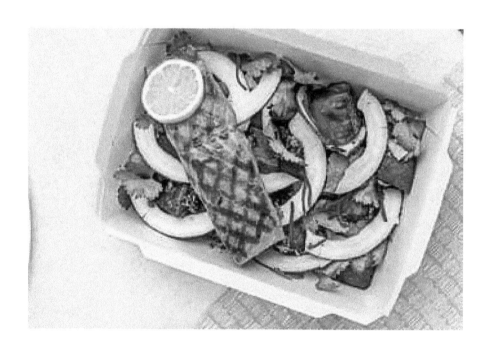

## © Copyright 2020 - All rights reserved.

The content contained within this book may not be reproduced, duplicated or transmitted without direct written permission from the author or the publisher.

Under no circumstances will any blame or legal responsibility be held against the publisher, or author, for any damages, reparation, or monetary loss due to the information contained within this book. Either directly or indirectly.

### Legal Notice:

This book is copyright protected. This book is only for personal use. You cannot amend, distribute, sell, use, quote or paraphrase any part, or the content within this book, without the consent of the author or publisher.

### Disclaimer Notice:

Please note the information contained within this document is for educational and entertainment purposes only. All effort has been executed to present accurate, up to date, and reliable, complete information. No warranties of any kind are declared or implied. Readers acknowledge that the author is not engaging in the rendering of legal, financial, medical or professional advice. The content within this book has been derived from various sources.

Please consult a licensed professional before attempting any techniques outlined in this book.

By reading this document, the reader agrees that under no circumstances is the author responsible for any losses, direct or indirect, which are incurred as a result of the use of information contained within this document, including, but not limited to, — errors, omissions, or inaccuracies.

# Table of contents

# Bacon Breakfast Bagels Bread

Preparation Time: 7 minutes

Cooking Time: 15 minutes

Servings: 8

Ingredients:

Bagels

- 3/4 cup (68 g) almond flour
- 1 teaspoon thickener
- 1 huge egg
- 1 1/2 cups ground mozzarella
- 2 tablespoons cream cheddar
- 1 tablespoon spread, softened
- Sesame seeds to taste

Fillings

- 2 tablespoons pesto
- 2 tablespoons cream cheddar
- 1 cup arugula leaves
- 6 cuts flame-broiled streaky bacon

Directions:

1. Preheat the stove to 390F.
2. In a bowl, merge the almond flour and thickener. At that point, gather the egg and blend it into a single unit until very much consolidated. Put in a safe spot. It will resemble a raw ball.

3. In a pot over medium-low heat, gradually melt the cream cheddar and mozzarella together and expel from heat once softened. This should be possible in the microwave also.

4. Add your softened cheddar blend to the almond flour blend and fold until all combined. The Mozzarella combine will stick in somewhat of a ball, yet don't stress, endure with it. It will all, in the long run, mix well. It's imperative to get the Xanthan gum fused through the cheddar blend. On the off chance that the mixture gets too extreme to even think about working, place in the microwave for 10-20 seconds to warm and rehash until you have something that looks like batter.

5. Split your mixture into 3 pieces and fold into round logs. On the off chance that you have a doughnut skillet place your logs into the container. If not, make hovers with each log and consolidate and place it on a prepared plate. Attempt to ensure you have decent circles. The other method to do this is to make a ball and level marginally on the heating plate and cut a hover out of the center if you have a little cutout.

6. Melt your margarine and brush over your bagels' highest point and sprinkle sesame seeds or your garnish of decision. The margarine should enable the seeds to stick. Garlic and onion powder or cheddar causes decent increments on the off chance that you have them for flavorful bagels.

7. Place bagels on the stove for around 18 minutes. Watch out for them. The tops ought to go brilliant dark-colored.

8. Take the bagels out of the stove and permit cooling.
9. If you like your bagels toasted, divide them down the middle the long way and put them back in the stove until somewhat brilliant and toasty.
10. Spread bagel with creamy cheddar, spread in pesto, includes a couple of arugula leaves, and top with your fresh bacon (or your filling of decision.)

Nutrition:

Cal: 90

Carbs: 4g

Net Carbs: 2.5 g

Fiber: 4.5 g

Fat: 8 g

Protein: 8g

Sugars: 3 g

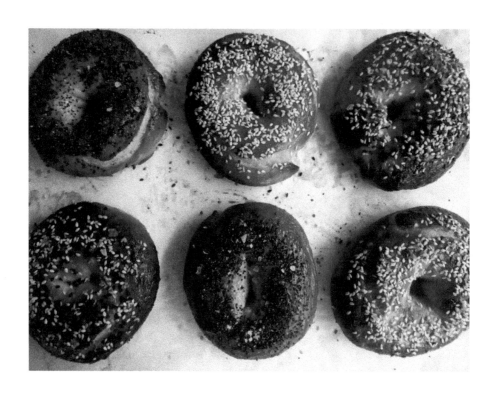

# Toast-Bread

Preparation Time: 3 1/2 hours

Cooking Time: 3 1/2 hours

Servings: 8

Ingredients:

- 1 1/2 teaspoons yeast
- 3 cups almond flour
- 2 tablespoons sugar
- 1 teaspoon salt
- 1 1/2 tablespoon butter
- 1 cup water

Directions:

1. Pour water into the bowl; add salt, sugar, soft butter, flour, and yeast.
2. I add dried tomatoes and paprika.
3. Put it on the basic program.
4. The crust can be light or medium.

Nutrition:

Cal: 203

Carbs: 5 g

Fats 2.7 g

Protein 5.2 g

Fiber: 1 g

# Lovely Oatmeal Bread

Preparation Time: 10 minutes or less

Cooking Time: 50 minutes

Servings: 8

Ingredients:

- 3/4 cup water, at 80F to 90F
- 2 tablespoons melted butter, cooled
- 2 tablespoons sugar
- 1 teaspoon salt
- 3/4 cup quick oats
- 11/2 cups white bread flour
- 1 teaspoon bread machine or instant yeast
- 12 slices / 11/2 pounds
- 11/8 cups water, at 80°F to 90°F
- 3 tablespoons melted butter, cooled
- 3 tablespoons sugar
- 11/2 teaspoons salt
- 1 cup quick oats
- 21/4 cups white bread flour
- 11/2 teaspoons bread machine or instant yeast
- 16 slices / 2 pounds
- 11/2 cups water, at 80°F to 90°F
- 1/4 cup melted butter, cooled
- 1/4 cup sugar
- 2 teaspoons salt

- 11/2 cups quick oats
- 3 cups flour
- 2 teaspoons yeast

Directions

1. Set the ingredients in your device.
2. Choose the machine for Basic/White bread, select light or medium crust, and choose Start.
3. When the loaf is done, remove the bucket from the machine.
4. Let the loaf cool.
5. Carefully shake the bucket to remove the loaf and turn it out onto a rack to cool.

Nutrition:

Cal: 149

Total fat: 4g

Saturated fat: 2g

Carbs: 26g

Fiber: 1g

Sodium: 312mg

Protein: 4g

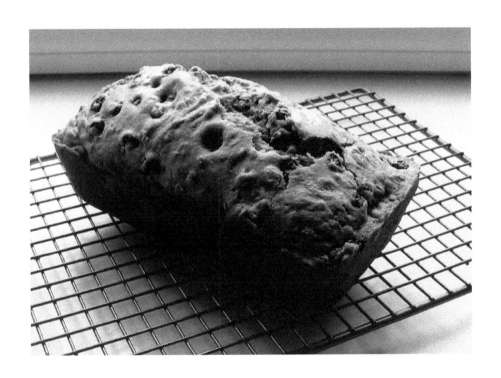

# Chicken Parmesan Chaffles

Preparation time: 10 minutes

Cooking Time: 8 Minutes

Servings: 2

Ingredients:

- 1/3 cup chicken
- 1 egg
- 1/3 cup mozzarella cheese
- 1/4 tsp. basil
- 1/4 garlic
- 2 tbsp. tomato sauce
- 2 tbsp. Mozzarella cheese

Directions:

1. Set up your Dash mini Chaffle maker device.
2. In a small bowl, merge the egg, Cooked chicken, basil, garlic, and Mozzarella Cheese.
3. Add 1/2 of the batter into your mini Chaffle maker and Cooking for 4 minutes. If they are still a bit cooked, leave it Cooking for another 2 minutes. Then Cooking the rest of the batter to make a second chaffle and then cook.
4. After Cooking, detach from the pan and let sit for 2 minutes.
5. Set with 1-2 tablespoons sauce on each chicken parmesan chaffle. Then set 1-2 tablespoon mozzarella cheese.

6. Set chaffles in the oven or a toaster oven at 400 degrees and Cooking until the cheese is melted.

Nutrition:

Calories 186

Protein 23 g

Fat 2g

Cholesterol 41 mg

Potassium 282 mg

Calcium 160 mg

Fiber 1.1 g

# Pork Tzatziki Chaffle

Preparation time: 10 minutes

Cooking Time: 25 Minutes

Servings: 2

Ingredients:

- 4 eggs
- 2 cups grated provolone cheese
- Salt and pepper to taste
- 1 teaspoon dried rosemary
- 1 teaspoon dried oregano
- 2 tablespoons olive oil
- 1 pound pork tenderloin
- Salt and pepper to taste
- Tzatziki sauce
- 1 cup sour cream
- Salt and pepper to taste
- 1 cucumber, peeled and diced
- 1 teaspoon garlic powder
- 1 teaspoon dried dill
- 2 tablespoons butter to brush the Chaffle maker

Directions:

1. Preheat the Chaffle maker.
2. Add the eggs, grated provolone cheese, dried rosemary, and dried oregano to a bowl. Season with salt and pepper to taste.

18

3. Mix until combined.
4. Brush the heated Chaffle maker with butter and add a few tablespoons of the batter.
5. Close the lid and Cooking for about 7 minutes depending on your Chaffle maker.
6. Meanwhile, heat the olive oil in a nonstick frying pan. Generously season the pork tenderloin with salt and pepper and Cook it for about 7 minutes on each side.
7. Mix the sour cream, salt and pepper, diced cucumber, garlic powder and dried dill in a bowl.
8. Serve each chaffle with a few tablespoons of tzatziki sauce and slices of pork tenderloin.

Nutrition:

Calories 104

Protein 6 g

Fat 4 g

Cholesterol 11 mg

Potassium 141 mg

Calcium 69 mg

Fiber 2.4 g

# Mediterranean Lamb Kebabs on Chaffles

Preparation time: 10 minutes

Cooking Time: 15 Minutes

Servings: 2

Ingredients:

- 4 eggs
- 2 cups grated mozzarella cheese
- Salt and pepper to taste
- 1 teaspoon garlic powder
- 1/4 cup Greek yogurt
- 1/2 cup coconut flour
- 2 teaspoons baking powder
- 1 pound ground lamb meat
- Salt and pepper to taste
- 1 egg
- 2 tablespoons almond flour
- 1 spring onion, finely chopped
- 1/2 teaspoon dried garlic
- 2 tablespoons olive oil
- 2 tablespoons butter to brush the Chaffle maker
- 1/4 cup sour cream for serving
- 4 sprigs of fresh dill for garnish

Directions:

1. Preheat the Chaffle maker.
2. Add the eggs, mozzarella cheese, salt and pepper, garlic powder, Greek yogurt, coconut flour and baking powder to a bowl.
3. Mix until combined.
4. Brush the heated Chaffle maker with butter and add a few tablespoons of the batter.
5. Close the lid and Cooking for about 7 minutes depending on your Chaffle maker.
6. Meanwhile, add the ground lamb, salt and pepper, egg, almond flour, chopped spring onion, and dried garlic to a bowl. Mix and form medium-sized kebabs.
7. Impale each kebab on a skewer. Warmth the olive oil in a frying pan.
8. Cooking the lamb kebabs for about 3 minutes on each side.
9. Serve each chaffle with a tablespoon of sour cream and one or two lamb kebabs. Decorate with fresh dill.

Nutrition:

Calories 132

Protein 10 g

Fat 0 g

Cholesterol 0 mg

Potassium 353 mg

Calcium 9 mg

Fiber 1.9 g

# Simple Beef and Sour Cream Chaffle

Preparation time: 10 minutes

Cooking Time: 15 Minutes

Servings: 2

Ingredients:

- 4 eggs
- 2 cups grated mozzarella cheese
- 3 tablespoons coconut flour
- 3 tablespoons almond flour
- 2 teaspoons baking powder
- Salt and pepper to taste
- 1 tablespoon freshly chopped parsley
- 1 pound beef tenderloin
- Salt and pepper to taste
- 2 tablespoons olive oil
- 1 tablespoon Dijon mustard
- 2 tablespoons olive oil to brush the Chaffle maker
- 1/4 cup sour cream for garnish
- 2 tablespoons freshly chopped spring onion for garnish

Directions:

1. Preheat the Chaffle maker.
2. Add the eggs, grated mozzarella cheese, coconut flour, almond flour, baking powder, salt and pepper and freshly chopped parsley to a bowl.
3. Mix until just combined and batter forms.

4. Brush the heated Chaffle maker with olive oil and add a few tablespoons of the batter.
5. Close the lid and Cooking for about 7 minutes depending on your Chaffle maker.
6. Meanwhile, heat the olive oil in a nonstick pan over medium heat.
7. Season the beef tenderloin with salt and pepper and spread the whole piece of beef tenderloin with Dijon mustard.
8. Cook on each side for about 45 minutes.
9. Serve each chaffle with sour cream and slices of the Cooked beef tenderloin.
10. Garnish with freshly chopped spring onion.
11. Serve and enjoy.

Nutrition:

Calories 126

Protein 12 g

Fat 0.03 g

Cholesterol 0 mg

Potassium 220 mg

Calcium 19 mg

Fiber 1.4g

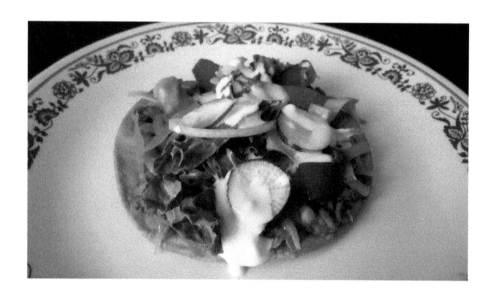

# Pork Loin Chaffles Sandwich

Preparation time: 10 minutes

Cooking Time: 15 Minutes

Servings: 2

Ingredients:

- 4 eggs
- 1 cup grated mozzarella cheese
- 1 cup grated parmesan cheese
- Salt and pepper to taste
- 2 tablespoons cream cheese
- 6 tablespoons coconut flour
- 2 teaspoons baking powder
- 2 tablespoons olive oil
- 1 pound pork loin
- Salt and pepper to taste
- 2 cloves garlic, minced
- 1 tablespoon freshly chopped thyme
- 2 tablespoons Cooking spray to brush the Chaffle maker
- 4 lettuce leaves for serving
- 4 slices of tomato for serving
- 1/4 cup sugar-free mayonnaise for serving

Directions:

1. Preheat the Chaffle maker.

2. Add the eggs, mozzarella cheese, parmesan cheese, salt and pepper, cream cheese, coconut flour and baking powder to a bowl.

3. Mix until combined.

4. Brush the heated Chaffle maker with Cooking spray and add a few tablespoons of the batter.

5. Close the lid and Cooking for about 7 minutes depending on your Chaffle maker.

6. Meanwhile, heat the olive oil in a nonstick frying pan and season the pork loin with salt and pepper, minced garlic and freshly chopped thyme.

7. Cooking the pork loin for about 5–minutes on each side.

8. Cut each chaffle in half and add some mayonnaise, lettuce leaf, tomato slice and sliced pork loin on one half.

9. Cover the sandwich with the other chaffle half and serve.

Nutrition:

Calories 141

Protein 10 g

Carbohydrates 15 g

Fat 0 g

Sodium 113 mg

# Beef Chaffles Tower

Preparation time: 10 minutes

Cooking Time: 15 Minutes

Servings: 2

Ingredients:

Batter

- 4 eggs
- 2 cups grated mozzarella cheese
- Salt and pepper to taste
- 2 tablespoons almond flour
- 1 teaspoon Italian seasoning
- 2 tablespoons butter
- 1 pound beef tenderloin
- Salt and pepper to taste
- 1 teaspoon chili flakes
- 2 tablespoons Cooking spray to brush the Chaffle maker

Directions:

1. Preheat the Chaffle maker.
2. Add the eggs, grated mozzarella cheese, salt and pepper, almond flour and Italian seasoning to a bowl.
3. Mix until everything is fully combined.
4. Brush the heated Chaffle maker with Cooking spray and add a few tablespoons of the batter.
5. Close the lid and Cooking for about 7 minutes depending on your Chaffle maker.

6. Meanwhile, heat the butter in a nonstick frying pan and season the beef tenderloin with salt and pepper and chili flakes.

7. Cooking the beef tenderloin for about 5–minutes on each side.

8. When serving, assemble the chaffle tower by placing one chaffle on a plate, a layer of diced beef tenderloin, another chaffle, another layer of beef, and so on until you finish with the chaffles and beef.

9. Serve and enjoy.

Nutrition:

Calories 132

Protein 9g

Carbohydrates 14 g

Sodium 112 mg

Potassium 310 mg,

Phosphorus 39 mg

Calcium 32 mg

# Ground Chicken and Turkey Chaffles

Preparation time: 10 minutes

Cooking Time: 1 hour 15 Minutes

Servings: 10

Ingredients:

- 8 ounces grass-fed ground chicken
- 8 ounces ground turkey
- 10 organic eggs
- 4 tablespoons Parmesan cheese, shredded
- 2 tablespoons organic baking powder
- 1/4 teaspoon cayenne pepper
- Salt and ground black pepper

Directions:

1. In a pan of water, cook the ground meats for about 8-10 minutes.
2. Remove from the heat and through a colander, drain the meat completely.
3. Set aside to cool for about 5 minutes.
4. In a bowl, add the cooked meats and remaining ingredients and mix well.
5. Preheat a mini Chaffle iron and then grease it.
6. In a medium bowl, set all ingredients and mix until well combined.
7. Divide the mixture into 10 portions.

8. Place 1 portion of the mixture into preheated Chaffle iron and cook for about 5-7 minutes or until golden brown.

9. Repeat with the remaining mixture.

10. Serve warm.

Nutrition:

Calories: 162

Net Carb: 1.8g

Fat: 9.1g

Carbohydrates: 1.9g

Dietary Fiber: 0.1g

Sugar: 0.4g

Protein: 19.1g

# Chicken and Ham Chaffles

Preparation Time: 10 minutes

Cooking Time: 16 minutes

Servings: 4

Ingredients:

- 1/4 cup grass-fed cooked chicken, chopped
- 1 ounce sugar-free ham, chopped
- 1 organic egg, beaten
- 1/4 cup Swiss cheese, shredded
- 1/4 cup Mozzarella cheese, shredded

Directions:

1. Preheat a mini Chaffle iron and then grease it.
2. In a medium bowl, set all ingredients and mix until well combined.
3. Place 1/4 of the mixture into preheated Chaffle iron and cook for about 4 minutes or until golden brown.
4. Repeat with the remaining mixture.
5. Serve warm.

Nutrition:

Calories: 71

Net Carb: 0.7g

Fat: 4.2g

Carbohydrates: 0.8g

Dietary Fiber: 0.1g

Sugar: 0.2g

Protein: 7.4g

# Chicken and Zucchini Chaffles

Preparation Time: 15 minutes

Cooking Time: 27 minutes

Servings: 9

Ingredients:

- 2 ounces cooked grass-fed chicken, chopped
- 1 cup zucchini, shredded and squeezed
- 2 tablespoons scallion, chopped
- 1 large organic egg
- 1/4 cup Mozzarella cheese, shredded
- 1/4 cup Cheddar cheese, shredded
- 1/4 cup blanched almond flour
- 1/2 teaspoon organic baking powder
- 1/4 teaspoon garlic salt
- 1/4 teaspoon onion powder

Directions:

1. Preheat a mini Chaffle iron and then grease it.
2. In a medium bowl, set all ingredients and mix until well combined.
3. Divide the mixture into 9 portions.
4. Place 1 portion of the mixture into preheated Chaffle iron and cook for about 2-3 minutes or until golden brown.
5. Repeat with the remaining mixture.
6. Serve warm.

Nutrition:

Calories: 64

Net Carb: 1g

Fat: 4.4g

Carbohydrates: 1.5g

Dietary Fiber: 0.5g

Sugar: 0.5g

Protein: 4.3g

# Chicken Chaffles with Tzatziki

Preparation Time: 15 minutes

Cooking Time: 12 minutes

Servings: 2

Ingredients:

Chaffles

- 1 organic egg, beaten
- 1/3 cup grass-fed cooked chicken, chopped
- 1/3 cup mozzarella cheese, shredded
- 1/4 teaspoon garlic, minced
- 1/4 teaspoon dried basil, crushed

Tzatziki

- 1/4 cup plain Greek yogurt
- 1/2 of small cucumber, peeled, seeded, and chopped
- 1 teaspoon olive oil
- 1/2 teaspoon fresh lemon juice
- Pinch of ground black pepper
- 1/4 tablespoon fresh dill, chopped
- 1/2 of garlic clove, peeled

Directions:

1. Preheat a mini Chaffle iron and then grease it.
2. For chaffles: In a medium bowl, put all ingredients and with your hands, mix until well merged. Place half of the mixture

into preheated Chaffle iron and cook for about 4–6 minutes.

3. Repeat with the remaining mixture.
4. Meanwhile, for tzatziki: in a food processor, place all the ingredients and pulse until well combined.
5. Serve warm chaffles alongside the tza tziki.

Nutrition:

Calories 131

Net Carbs 4.4

Total Fat 5 g

Saturated Fat 2 g

Cholesterol 104 mg

Sodium 97 mg

Total Carbs 4.7 g

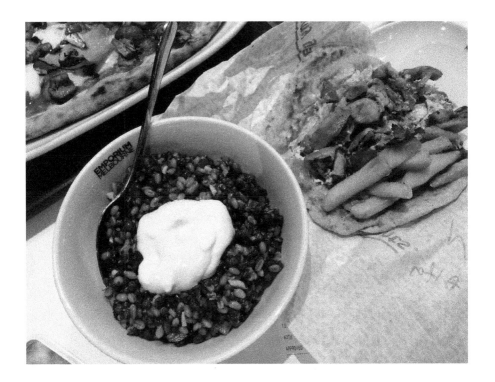

# Keema Curry Chaffle

Preparation time: 10 minutes

Cooking time: 10 minutes

Servings: 4

Ingredients:

- 2 eggs
- 3 oz. mozzarella cheese, shredded
- 3 tbsp. almond flour
- 1/2 tsp. baking powder
- 1/4 tsp. garlic powder
  - oz. ground beef
- 1 tbsp. avocado oil
- 1/4 tsp. salt
- 1/2 tsp. garlic powder
- 1/4 tsp. ginger powder
- 1/2 cup tomato puree
- 2 tbsp. curry powder
- 2 tbsp. Worcestershire sauce
- 4 tsp. parmesan cheese, finely grated

Directions:

1. Start by making the curry, over medium heat, heat avocado oil in a frying pan.
2. Add in the ground meat and Cooking until it turns brown.
3. Add the ginger powder, garlic powder, and salt. Stir well.
4. Stir in the Worcestershire sauce and the tomato puree.

5. Finally, add the curry powder and stir it in.
6. Allow to simmer for about 6-10 minutes over low heat.
7. Preheat the mini Chaffle maker.
8. Combine all chaffle ingredients, except cheese, in a small mixing bowl.
9. Sprinkle some cheese onto the heated Chaffle maker and let it melt.
10. When the cheese melts, immediately pour 1/4 of the batter on top of it. Spread 2 tsp. of keema curry then sprinkle some more cheese.
11. Close the lid. Cooking for 4 minutes.
12. Remove the cooked chaffle and repeat the steps until you've used up all the batter.
13. Once all chaffles are cooked, use the remaining keema curry on top.
14. Top all the chaffles with parmesan cheese.

Nutrition:

Calories: 374

Carbohydrate: 8g

Fat: 25g

Protein: 27g

# Delicious Carrot Cake

Preparation Time: 15 minutes

Cooking Time: 55 minutes

Servings: 6

Ingredients

- 2 large eggs
- 1/2 cup carrots, grated
- 1 tsp. vanilla
- 2 tbsp. coconut oil, melted
- 3 tbsp. heavy cream
- 1/4 tsp. nutmeg
- 1/2 tsp. cinnamon
- 1 tsp. baking powder
- 2/3 cup Swerve
- 1 cup almond flour

For Frosting:

- 1 tbsp. heavy cream
- 1/2 tsp. vanilla
- 2 tsp. fresh lemon juice
- 3 tbsp. swerve
- 4 oz. cream cheese, softened

Direction

1. Take a cake pan which fits into the instant pot and spray with Cooking spray and set aside.

2. Drain excess liquid from grated carrots.
3. In a mixing bowl, merge together almond flour, grated carrots, vanilla, coconut oil, heavy cream, eggs, nutmeg, cinnamon, baking powder, and swerve using a hand mixer until well combined.
4. Pour batter into the prepare cake pan and cover the pan with foil.
5. Add 1 2/3 cup of water to the instant pot then place steamer rack into the pot.
6. Place cake pan on the steamer rack.
7. Seal instant pot with lid and select manual high pressure and set the timer for 45 minutes.
8. Set to release pressure naturally for 10 minutes then release using the quick release method.
9. Open the lid carefully and remove cake pan from the pot. Let the cake cool for 30 minutes.
10. Meanwhile, make the frosting. In a large bowl add heavy cream, vanilla, lemon juice, swerve, and cream cheese and beat using a hand mixer until creamy.
11. Once the cake is cool completely then frost cake using prepared cream.
12. Cut cake into the slices and serve.

Nutrition:

Calories 289

Fat 25.9 g

Carbohydrates 10.9 g

Sugar 1.5 g

Protein 7.9 g

Cholesterol 97 mg

# Almond Coconut Cake

Preparation Time: 10 minutes

Cooking Time: 50 minutes

Servings: 8

Ingredients

- 2 eggs, lightly beaten
- 1/2 cup heavy cream
- 1/4 cup coconut oil, melted
- 1 tsp. cinnamon
- 1 tsp. baking powder
- 1/3 cup Swerve
- 1/2 cup unsweetened shredded coconut
- 1 cup almond flour

Direction

1. Spray a 6- inch cake pan with Cooking spray and set aside.
2. In a large bowl, mix together the almond flour, cinnamon, baking powder, swerve, and shredded coconut.
3. Add eggs, heavy cream, and coconut oil into the almond flour mixture and mix until well combined.
4. Pour batter into the prepare cake pan and cover the pan with foil.
5. Attach 2 cups of water into the instant pot then place a steamer rack in the pot.
6. Place cake pan on top of steamer rack.

7. Seal instant pot with lid and select manual high pressure and set the timer for 40 minutes.
8. Once the timer goes off then allows to release pressure naturally for 10 minutes then release using quick release method.
9. Open the lid carefully. Remove cake pan from the pot and let it cool for 20 minutes.
10. Cut cake into the slices and serve.

Nutrition:

Calories 228

Fat 21.7 g

Carbohydrates 5.2 g

Sugar 1.2 g

Protein 5 g

Cholesterol 51 mg

# Tasty Chocolate Cake

Preparation Time: 10 minutes

Cooking Time: 30 minutes

Servings: 6

Ingredients

- 3 large eggs
- 1/4 cup butter, melted
- 1/3 cup heavy cream
- 1 tsp. baking powder
- 1/4 cup walnuts, chopped
- 1/4 cup unsweetened cocoa powder
- 2/3 cup Swerve
- 1 cup almond flour

Direction

1. Set cake pan with Cooking spray and set aside.
2. Add all ingredients into a large mixing bowl and mix using a hand mixer until the mixture looks fluffy.
3. Pour batter into the prepared cake pan.
4. Set 2 cups of water into the instant pot then place a steamer rack in the pot.
5. Place cake pan on top of steamer rack.
6. Seal instant pot with lid and Cooking on manual high pressure for 20 minutes.
7. Set to release pressure naturally for 10 minutes then release using the quick release method.

8. Open the lid carefully. Remove cake pan from the pot and let it cool for 20 minutes.
9. Cut cake into the slices and serve.

Nutrition:

Calories 275

Fat 25.5 g

Carbohydrates 7.5 g

Sugar 1 g

Protein 9.3 g

Cholesterol 122 mg

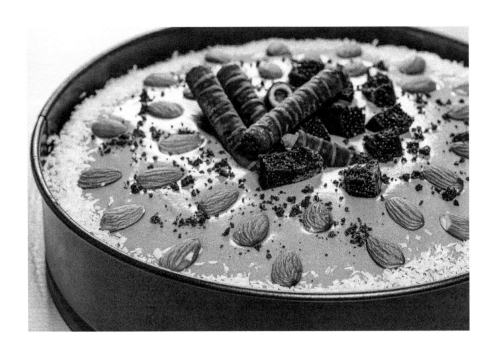

# Almond Spice Cake

Preparation Time: 10 minutes

Cooking Time: 55 minutes

Servings: 10

Ingredients

- 2 large eggs
- 2 cups almond flour
- 3 tbsp. walnuts (or pistachios), chopped
- 1/2 tsp. vanilla
- 1/3 cup water
- 1/3 cup coconut oil, melted
- 1/4 tsp. ground cloves
- 1 tsp. ground ginger
- 1 tsp. cinnamon
- 2 tsp. baking powder
- 1/2 cup Swerve
- Pinch of salt

DIRECTION

1. Spray 7-inch cake pan with Cooking spray and set aside.
2. Set 1 cup of water into the instant pot then place a trivet in the pot.
3. In a mixing bowl, whisk together the almond flour, cloves, ginger, cinnamon, baking powder, salt and swerve.
4. Stir in the eggs, vanilla, water, and coconut oil until combined.

5. Set batter into the cake pan and sprinkle chopped walnuts (or pistachios) on top. Cover the cake pan with foil and place on top of trivet in the instant pot.
6. Seal pot with lid and Cooking on manual high pressure for 40 minutes.
7. Set to release pressure naturally for 15 minutes. Open the lid carefully.
8. Remove cake pan from the pot and let it cool for 20 minutes.
9. Cut cake into the slices and serve.

Nutrition:

Calories 223

Fat 20.9 g

Carbohydrates 6.1 g

Sugar 0.9 g

Protein 6.7 g

Cholesterol 37 mg

# Walnut Carrot Cake

Preparation Time: 10 minutes

Cooking Time: 50 minutes

Servings: 8

Ingredients

- 3 large eggs
- 1/2 cup walnuts, chopped
- 1 cup carrots, shredded
- 1/2 cup heavy cream
- 1/4 cup butter, melted
- 1 1/2 tsp. apple pie spice
- 1 tsp. baking powder
- 2/3 cup Swerve
- 1 cup almond flour

Direction

1. Set a 6-inch cake pan with Cooking spray and set aside.
2. Add all ingredients into the large mixing bowl and mix using a hand mixer until mixture is well combined and looks fluffy.
3. Pour batter into the cake pan and cover the pan with foil.
4. Set 2 cups of water into the instant pot then place a trivet in the pot.
5. Set cake pan on top of the trivet.
6. Seal pot with lid and Cooking on manual high pressure for 40 minutes.

7. Allow to release pressure naturally
8. Open the lid carefully. Remove cake pan from the pot and let it cool for 20 minutes.
9. Slice and serve.

Nutrition:

Calories 240

Fat 22 g

Carbohydrates 6.2 g

Sugar 1.4 g

Protein 7.6 g

Cholesterol 95 mg

# Cinnamon Almond Butter Cake

Preparation Time: 10 minutes

Cooking Time: 35 minutes

Servings: 8

Ingredients

- 2 large eggs
- 1/4 tsp. apple pie spice
- 1/4 tsp. cinnamon
- 1 tbsp. unsweetened cocoa powder
- 1/2 cup cream cheese
- 1/4 cup almond butter
- 1/2 cup Swerve
- 1/2 cup almond, minced
- 1 cup coconut flour
- Pinch of salt

Direction

1. In a large bowl, merge together the coconut flour, apple pie spice, cinnamon, swerve, almonds, and salt until well combined.
2. Slowly, add the eggs, cream cheese, and almond butter and beat using a hand mixer until combined.
3. Set 1 cup of water into the instant pot then place a trivet in the pot.
4. Line spring form pan with parchment paper.

5. Set the batter into the pan and spread evenly. Cover the pan with foil and place on top of the trivet in the instant pot.
6. Seal pot with lid and Cooking on manual high pressure for 35 minutes.
7. Remove cake pan from the pot and let it cool for 30 minutes.
8. Sprinkle cocoa powder or chopped almonds on top of the cake.
9. Slice and serve.

Nutrition:

Calories 116

Fat 9.9 g

Carbohydrates 3.4 g

Sugar 0.5 g

Protein 4.4 g

Cholesterol 62 mg

# Healthy Almond Bars

Preparation Time: 10 minutes

Cooking Time: 25 minutes

Servings: 6

Ingredients

- 2 large eggs
- 1/2 tsp. vanilla
- 2 1/2 tbsp. swerve
- 2 tbsp. almond butter
- 1/2 cup of coconut oil
- 1/4 cup coconut flour
- 1 1/2 cup almond flour
- Pinch of salt

Direction

1. Set 1 cup of water into the instant pot then place a trivet in the pot.
2. Add all the ingredients into a food processor and process until well combined.
3. Take one baking pan which fits into your instant pot. Line the baking pan with parchment paper.
4. Add dough to the pan and spread dough gently with the palm of your hands.
5. Place baking pan on top of trivet in the instant pot.
6. Seal instant pot with lid and select manual and set the timer for 15 minutes.

7. Set to release pressure naturally for 10 minutes then release using the quick release method.
8. Open the lid carefully. Remove baking pan from the instant pot and let it cool for 20 minutes.
9. Slice into bars and place in refrigerator for 1-2 hours.

Nutrition:

Calories 379

Fat 36.9 g

Carbohydrates 8.3 g

Sugar 1.4 g

Protein 9.3 g

Cholesterol 62 mg

# Dark Chocolate Bars

Preparation Time: 10 minutes

Cooking Time: 12 minutes

Servings: 4

Ingredients

- 1 large egg
- 1 tsp. stevia
- 1/2 cup unsweetened dark chocolate, grated
- 1 tbsp. unsweetened cocoa powder
- 1/2 cup almond butter
- 1/2 cup unsweetened almond milk
- 1 tsp. vanilla
- 2 cups almond flour

Direction

1. Pour 2 cups of water into the instant pot then place a trivet in the pot.
2. Line a baking dish with parchment paper and set aside.
3. Add all ingredients into the food processor and process until smooth.
4. Transfer mixture into the prepared baking dish and spread evenly with your hands.
5. Cover baking dish with foil and place on top of trivet in the instant pot.
6. Seal the instant pot with lid and select manual and set the timer for 12 minutes.

7. Release pressure using the quick release method than open the lid.

8. Remove baking dish from the instant pot and let it cool for 20 minutes.

9. Cut bar into slices and place in refrigerator for 1-2 hours.

Nutrition:

Calories 321

Fat 26 g

Carbohydrates 13 g

Sugar 0.8 g

Protein 9.4 g

Cholesterol 47 mg

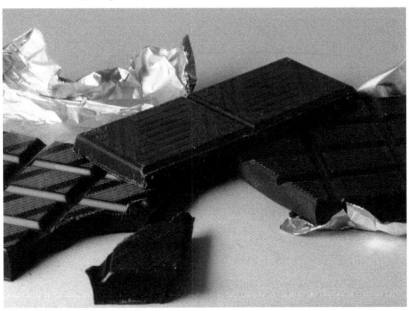

# Coconut Bars

Preparation Time: 10 minutes

Cooking Time: 15 minutes

Servings: 6

Ingredients

- 3 large eggs
- 1 tsp. vanilla
- 2 cups shredded coconut
- 1/4 cup almonds, chopped
- 1 tbsp. chia seeds
- 2 tbsp. swerve
- 2 tbsp. almond butter
- 1/2 cup of coconut oil
- 1/4 cup flaxseed meal
- Pinch of salt

Direction

1. Pour 2 cups of water into the instant pot then place a trivet in the pot.
2. Line a baking pan with parchment paper and set aside.
3. Add all ingredients into the large mixing bowl and mix until the mixture is sticky.
4. Add the mixture to the baking pan and spread evenly with the palms of your hands.
5. Cover baking pan with foil and place on top of trivet in the instant pot.

6. Seal pot with lid and select manual and set timer for 15 minutes.
7. Release pressure using the quick release method then open the lid.
8. Cut the bar into slices and place in refrigerator for 1-2 hours.

Nutrition:

Calories 376

Fat 36.4 g

Carbohydrates 8.4 g

Sugar 2.4 g

Protein 7.2 g

Cholesterol 93 mg

# Chia Nut Bars

Preparation Time: 10 minutes

Cooking Time: 25 minutes

Servings: 10

Ingredients

- 1 cup almond butter
- 2 1/2 tbsp. swerve
- 2 tbsp. chia seeds
- 1/4 tsp. cinnamon
- 1/2 cup almond flour
- 1/4 cup unsweetened cocoa powder
- 1/4 cup hazelnuts, chopped
- 1 cup almonds, chopped
- Pinch of salt

Direction

1. Line a baking dish with parchment paper and set aside.
2. Set 1 cup of water into the instant pot and place trivet in the pot.
3. Add the almond butter, swerve, cinnamon, almond flour, cocoa powder, hazelnuts, almonds, and salt into the food processor and process until smooth.
4. Transfer mixture into the large bowl. Add chia seeds and mix well.
5. Transfer mixture into the prepared baking dish and spread mixture evenly.

6. Cover baking dish with foil and place on top of trivet in the instant pot.
7. Seal pot with lid and select manual and set timer for 15 minutes.
8. Set to release pressure naturally for 10 minutes then release using the quick release method.
9. Open the lid carefully. Remove baking dish from the instant pot and let it cool for 20 minutes.
10. Cut the bar into slices and serve.

Nutrition:

Calories 122

Fat 10.3 g

Carbohydrates 5.9 g

Sugar 0.8 g

Protein 4.6 g

Cholesterol 0 mg

# Bagel Seasoning Chaffles

Preparation Time: 15 minutes

Cooking Time: 20 minutes

Servings: 4

Ingredients

- 1 large organic egg
- 1 cup Mozzarella cheese, shredded
- 1 tablespoon almond flour
- 1 teaspoon organic baking powder
- 2 teaspoons bagel seasoning
- 1/4 teaspoon garlic powder
- 1/4 teaspoon onion powder

Directions:

1. Preheat a mini Chaffle iron and then grease it.
2. In a medium bowl, set all ingredients and with a fork, mix until well combined.
3. Place 1/4 of the mixture into preheated Chaffle iron and Cooking for about 4 minutes or until golden brown.
4. Repeat with the remaining mixture.
5. Serve warm.

Nutrition:

Calories: 73

Net Carb: 2g

Fat: 5.5g

Saturated Fat: 1.5g

Carbohydrates: 2.3g

Dietary Fiber: 0.3g

Sugar: 0.9g

Protein: 3.7g

# Grilled Cheese Chaffle

Preparation Time: 5 minutes

Cooking Time: 10 minutes

Servings: 1

Ingredients

- 1 large egg
- 1/2 cup mozzarella cheese
- 2 slices yellow American cheese
- 2-3 slices Cooked bacon, cut in half
- 1 tsp. butter
- 1/2 tsp. baking powder

Directions:

1. Turn on Chaffle maker to heat and oil it with Cooking spray.
2. Beat egg in a bowl.
3. Add mozzarella, and baking powder.
4. Set half of the mix into the Chaffle maker and Cooking for minutes.
5. Remove and repeat to make the second chaffle.
6. Layer bacon and cheese slices in between two chaffles.
7. Melt butter in a skillet and add chaffle sandwich to the pan. Fry on each side for 2-3 minutes covered, until cheese has melted.
8. Divide in half on a plate and serve.

Nutrition:

Carbs: 4 g

Fat: 18 g

Protein: 7 g

Calories: 233

# Bbq Rub Chaffles

Preparation Time: 5 minutes

Cooking Time: 20 minutes

Servings: 4

Ingredients

- 2 organic eggs, beaten
- 1 cup Cheddar cheese, shredded
- 1/2 teaspoon BBQ rub
- 1/4 teaspoon organic baking powder

Directions:

1. Preheat a mini Chaffle iron and then grease it.
2. In a medium bowl, set all ingredients and with a fork, mix until well combined.
3. Place 1/4 of the mixture into preheated Chaffle iron and Cooking for about 5 minutes or until golden brown.
4. Repeat with the remaining mixture.
5. Serve warm.

Nutrition:

Calories: 14

Carb: 0.7g

Fat: 11.6g

Saturated Fat: 6.6g

Dietary Fiber: 0g

Sugar: 0.3g

Protein: 9.8g

# Pandan Asian Chaffles

Preparation Time: 5 minutes

Cooking Time: 8 minutes

Servings: 2

Ingredients

- 1/2 cup cheddar cheese, finely shredded
- 1 egg
- 3 drops of pandan extract
- 1 tbsp. almond flour
- 1/3 tsp. garlic powder

Directions:

1. Warm up your mini Chaffle maker.
2. Mix the egg, almond flour, garlic powder with cheese in a small bowl.
3. Add pandan extract to the cheese mixture and mix well.
4. For a crispy crust, add a teaspoon of shredded cheese to the Chaffle maker and Cooking for 30 seconds.
5. Then, set the mixture into the Chaffle maker and Cooking for minutes or until crispy.
6. Repeat with remaining batter.
7. Serve with fried chicken wings with bbq sauce and enjoy!

Nutrition:

Calories: 170

Fats: 13 g

Carbs: 2 g

Protein: 11 g

# Ham Chaffles

Preparation Time: 5 minutes

Cooking Time: 16 minutes

Servings: 4

Ingredients

- 2 large organic eggs (yolks and whites separated)
- 6 tablespoons butter, melted
- 2 scoops unflavored whey protein powder
- 1 teaspoon organic baking powder
- Salt, to taste
- 1 ounce sugar-free ham, chopped finely
- 1 ounce Cheddar cheese, shredded
- 1/8 teaspoon paprika

Directions:

1. Preheat a Chaffle iron and then grease it.
2. In a bowl place egg yolks, butter, protein powder, baking powder and salt and beat until well combined.
3. Add the ham steak pieces, cheese and paprika and stir to combine.
4. In another bowl, place 2 egg whites and a pinch of salt and with an electric hand mixer and beat until stiff peaks form.
5. Gently set the whipped egg whites into the egg yolk mixture in 2 batches.
6. Place 1/4 of the mixture into preheated Chaffle iron and Cooking for about 3-4 minutes or until golden brown.

7. Repeat with the remaining mixture.
8. Serve warm.

Nutrition:

Calories: 288

Net Carb: 1.5g

Fat: 22.8g

Saturated Fat: 13.4g

Carbohydrates: 1.7g

Dietary Fiber: 0.2g

Sugar: 0.3g

Protein: 20.3g

# Almond Taco Chaffles

Preparation Time: 5 minutes

Cooking Time: 20 minutes

Servings: 2

Ingredients

- 1 tablespoon almond flour
- 1 cup taco blend cheese
- 2 organic eggs
- 1/4 teaspoon taco seasoning

Directions:

1. Preheat a mini Chaffle iron and then grease it.
2. In a bowl, place all ingredients and mix until well combined.
3. Place 1/4 of the mixture into preheated Chaffle iron and Cooking for about 4 minutes or until golden brown.
4. Repeat with the remaining mixture.
5. Serve warm.

Nutrition:

Calories: 79

Net Carb: 0.7g

Fat: 5.4g

Saturated Fat: 2.2g

Carbohydrates: 0.9g

Dietary Fiber: 0.2g

Sugar: 0.3g

Protein: 4.5g

# Spinach and Cauliflower Chaffles

Preparation Time: 5 minutes

Cooking Time: 10 minutes

Servings: 2

Ingredients

- 1/2 cup frozen chopped spinach
- 1/2 cup cauliflower, chopped finely
- 1/2 cup Cheddar cheese, shredded
- 1/2 cup Mozzarella cheese, shredded
- 1/3 cup Parmesan cheese, , shredded
- 2 organic eggs
- 1 tablespoon butter, melted
- 1 teaspoon garlic powder
- 1 teaspoon onion powder
- Salt and freshly ground black pepper

Directions:

1. Preheat a Chaffle iron and then grease it.
2. In a medium bowl, set all ingredients and, mix until well combined.
3. Set half of the mixture into preheated Chaffle iron and Cooking for about 4-5 minutes or until golden brown.
4. Repeat with the remaining mixture.
5. Serve warm.

Nutrition:

Calories: 320

Net Carb: 4g

Fat: 24.5g

Saturated Fat: 14g

Carbohydrates: 5g

Dietary Fiber: 1g

Sugar: 1.9g

Protein: 20.8g

# Rosemary Chaffles

Preparation Time: 5 minutes

Cooking Time: 8 minutes

Servings: 2

Ingredients

- 1 organic egg, beaten
- 1/2 cup Cheddar cheese, shredded
- 1 tablespoon almond flour
- 1 tablespoon fresh rosemary, chopped
- Salt and freshly ground black pepper

Directions:

1. Preheat a mini Chaffle iron and then grease it.
2. For chaffles: In a medium bowl, place all ingredients and with a fork, mix until well merged.
3. Set half of the mixture into preheated Chaffle iron and Cooking for about 4 minutes or until golden brown.
4. Repeat with the remaining mixture.
5. Serve warm.

Nutrition:

Calories: 173

Net Carb: 1.1g

Fat: 13.7g

Saturated Fat: 9g

Carbohydrates: 2.2g

Dietary Fiber: 1.1g

Sugar: 0.4g

Protein: 9.9g

# Mango and Berries Chaffles

Preparation time: 10 minutes

Cooking time: 10 minutes

Servings: 4

Ingredients:

- 1/2 cup mango, peeled and cubed
- 1 cup blueberries
- 1 cup almond flour
- 1/2 cup cream cheese, soft
- 2 eggs, whisked
- 1 tablespoon heavy cream
- 1 teaspoon baking powder
- 3 tablespoons cashew butter

Directions:

1. Incorporate mango with the berries and the other ingredients and whisk well.
2. Pour 1/4 of the batter in the Chaffle iron, cook for 7 minutes and set to a plate.
3. Serve the chaffles warm.

Nutrition:

Calories 200

Fat 3g

Protein 11g

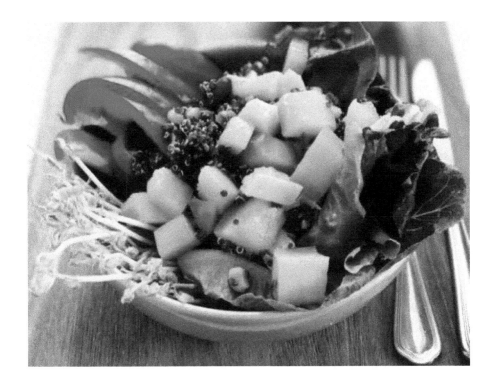

# Cauliflower Turmeric Buns

Preparation Time: 30 minutes

Cooking Time: 30 minutes

Servings: 6

Ingredients

- 1/4 tsp. ground turmeric
- 1 medium cauliflower head
- 2 eggs
- 2 Tbsp. coconut flour
- pinch of salt and pepper

Directions

1. Warmth the oven to 400F and line a baking sheet with parchment paper.
2. Pulse the cauliflower in a food processor until rice.
3. Add the rice cauliflower into a bowl with a tsp. of water, and then cover with a plastic wrap with some holes on top.
4. Place the cauliflower bowl into the microwave and heat for 4 minutes.
5. Remove the plastic wrap and cool the cauliflower for 5 minutes. Then transfer into paper towels and squeeze out all excess moisture.
6. Pour the squeezed cauliflower into a bowl. Add eggs, flour, turmeric, salt, pepper, and mix.
7. Mold the mixture into 6 buns, then arrange on top of the baking sheet and fit into the oven.

8. Bake for 25 to 30 minutes.

9. Serve.

Nutrition:

Calories: 65

Fat: 2.2g

Carb: 7.9g

Protein: 4.4g

# Salmon Chaffles

Preparation time: 6 minutes

Cooking Time: 10 Minutes

Servings: 2

Ingredients:

- 1 large egg
- 1/2 cup shredded mozzarella
- 1 Tbsp. cream cheese
- 2 slices salmon
- 1 Tbsp. everything bagel seasoning

Directions:

1. Turn on Chaffle maker to heat and oil it with Cooking spray.
2. Beat egg in a container, and then add 1/2 cup mozzarella.
3. Set half of the mixture into the Chaffle maker and Cooking for 4 minutes.
4. Remove and repeat with remaining mixture.
5. Let chaffles cool, then spread cream cheese, sprinkle with seasoning, and top with salmon.

Nutrition:

Carbs: 3 g

Fat: 10 g

Protein: 5 g

Calories: 201

# Chaffle Bruschetta

Preparation time: 5 minutes

Cooking Time: 5 Minutes

Servings: 2

Ingredients:

- 1/2 cup shredded mozzarella cheese
- 1 whole egg beaten
- 1/4 cup grated Parmesan cheese
- 1 tsp. Italian Seasoning
- 1/4 tsp. garlic powder

For the toppings:

- 3-4 cherry tomatoes, chopped
- 1 tsp. fresh basil, chopped
- Splash of olive oil
- Pinch of salt

Directions:

1. Turn on Chaffle maker to heat and oil it with Cooking spray.
2. Whisk all chaffle ingredients, except mozzarella, in a container.
3. Add in cheese and mix.
4. Add batter to Chaffle maker and Cooking for 5 minutes.
5. Mix tomatoes, basil, olive oil, and salt. Serve over the top of chaffleo.

Nutrition:

Carbs: 2 g

Fat: 24 g

Protein: 34 g

Calories: 352

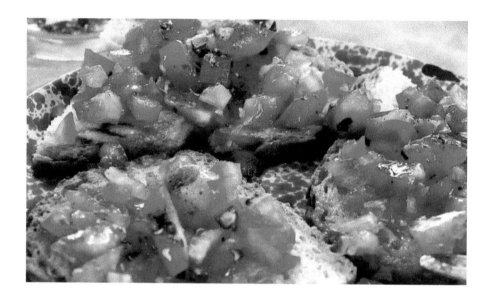

# Cheddar Protein Chaffles

Preparation time: 5 minutes

Cooking Time: 40 Minutes

Servings: 8

Ingredients:

- 1/2 cup golden flax seeds meal
- 1/2 cup almond flour
- 2 tablespoons unsweetened whey protein powder
- 1 teaspoon organic baking powder
- Salt and pepper, to taste
- 3/4 cup Cheddar cheese, shredded
- 1/3 cup unsweetened almond milk
- 2 tablespoons unsalted butter, melted
- 2 large organic eggs, beaten

Directions:

1. Preheat a mini Chaffle iron and then grease it.
2. In a large container, add flax seeds meal, flour, protein powder and baking powder and mix well.
3. Stir in the Cheddar cheese.
4. In another container, add the remaining ingredients and beat until well combined.
5. Add the egg mixture into the container with flax seeds meal mixture and mix until well combined.

6. Add desired amount of the mixture into preheated Chaffle iron and Cooking for about 4-5 minutes or until golden brown.
7. Repeat with the remaining mixture.
8. Serve warm.

Nutrition:

Calories: 187

Net Carb: 1.8g

Fat: 14.5g

Saturated Fat: 5g

Carbohydrates: 4.

Dietary Fiber: 3.1g

Sugar: 0.4g

Protein: 8g

# Eggs Benedict Chaffle

Preparation time: 6 minutes

Cooking Time: 10 Minutes

Servings: 2

Ingredients

For the chaffle:

- 2 egg whites
- 2 Tbsp. almond flour
- 1 Tbsp. sour cream
- 1/2 cup mozzarella cheese

For the hollandaise:

- 1/2 cup salted butter
- 4 egg yolks
- 2 Tbsp. lemon juice
- For the poached eggs:
- 2 eggs
- 1 Tbsp. white vinegar
- 3 oz. deli ham

Directions:

1. Whip egg white until frothy, and then mix in remaining ingredients.
2. Turn on Chaffle maker to heat and oil it with Cooking spray.
3. Cooking for 7 minutes until golden brown.
4. Remove chaffle and repeat with remaining batter.

5. Fill half the pot with water and bring to a boil.

6. Add heat-safe container on top of pot, ensuring bottom doesn't touch the boiling water.

7. Heat butter to boiling in a microwave.

8. Add yolks to double boiler container and bring to boil.

9. Add hot butter to the container and whisk briskly. Cooking until the egg yolk mixture has thickened.

10. Remove container from pot and add in lemon juice. Set aside.

11. Add more water to pot if needed to make the poached eggs (water should completely cover the eggs). Bring to a simmer. Add white vinegar to water.

12. Crack eggs into simmering water and Cooking for 1 minute 30 seconds. Remove using slotted spoon.

13. Warm chaffles in toaster for 2-3 minutes. Top with ham, poached eggs, and hollandaise sauce.

Nutrition:

Carbs: 4 g

Fat: 26 g

Protein: 26 g

Calories: 365

# Chicken Bacon Chaffle

Preparation time: 6 minutes

Cooking Time: 5 Minutes

Servings: 2

Ingredients:

- 1 egg
- 1/3 cup Cooked chicken, diced
- 1 piece of bacon, Cooked and crumbled
- 1/3 cup shredded cheddar jack cheese
- 1 tsp. powdered ranch dressing

Directions:

1. Turn on Chaffle maker to heat and oil it with Cooking spray.
2. Mix egg, dressing, and Monterey cheese in a container.
3. Add bacon and chicken.
4. Attach some of the batter to the Chaffle maker and Cooking for 3-minutes.
5. Remove and Cooking remaining batter to make a second chaffle.
6. Let chaffles sit for 2 minutes before serving.

Nutrition:

Carbs: 2 g;

Fat: 14 g;

Protein: 16 g

Calories: 200

# Garlicky Steaks with Rosemary

Preparation Time: 25 minutes

Cooking Time: 12 minutes

Servings: 2

Ingredients

- 2 beef steaks
- 1/4 of a lime, juiced
- 1 1/2 tsp. garlic powder
- 3/4 tsp. dried rosemary
- 2 1/2 tbsp. avocado oil

Seasoning:

- 1/2 tsp. salt
- 1/4 tsp. ground black pepper

Directions:

1. Prepare steaks, and for this, sprinkle garlic powder on all sides of steak.
2. Take a shallow dish, place 1 1/2 tbsp. oil and lime juice in it, whisk until combined, add steaks, turn to coat and let it marinate for 20 minutes at room temperature.
3. Then take a griddle pan, place it over medium-high heat and grease it with remaining oil.
4. Season marinated steaks with salt and black pepper; add to the griddle pan and Cooking for 7 to 12 minutes until cooked to the desired level.

5. When done, wrap steaks in foil for 5 minutes, and then cut into slices across the grain.

6. Sprinkle rosemary over steaks slices and then serve.

Nutrition:

Calories: 213

Fats: 13 g

Protein: 22 g

Net Carb: 1 g

Fiber: 0 g

# Rib Eye Steak

Preparation Time: 5 Minutes

Cooking Time: 20 Minutes

Servings: 2

Ingredients:

- 1/2 pound grass-fed rib-eye steak, preferably 1" thick
- 1 teaspoon Adobo Seasoning
- 1 tablespoon extra-virgin olive oil
- Pepper and sea salt to taste

Direction:

1. Add steak in a large-sized mixing bowl and drizzle both sides with a small amount of olive oil. Dust the seasonings on both sides; rubbing the seasonings into the meat.
2. Let sit for a couple of minutes and heat up your grill in advance. Once hot; place the steaks over the grill and Cooking until both sides are cooked through, for 15 to 20 minutes, flipping occasionally.

Nutrition:

Calories: 258

Fat: 19 g

Carbs: 5 g

Protein: 8 g

Fiber: 8 g

# Ground Beef and Green Beans

Preparation Time: 5 Minutes

Cooking Time: 10 Minutes

Servings: 2

Ingredients:

- 1 1/2 oz. butter
- 8 oz. green beans, fresh, rinsed, and trimmed
- 10 oz. ground beef
- 1/4 cup Crème Fraiche or home-made mayonnaise, optional
- Pepper and salt to taste

Direction:

1. Set moderate heat in a large frying pan; heat a generous dollop of butter until completely melted.
2. Increase the heat to high and immediately brown the ground beef until almost done, for 5 minutes. Sprinkle with pepper and salt to taste.
3. Decrease the heat to medium; add more of butter and continue to fry the beans in the same pan with the meat for 5 more minutes, stirring frequently.
4. Season the beans with pepper and salt as well. Serve with the leftover butter and add in the optional Crème Fraiche or mayonnaise, if desired.

Nutrition:

Calories: 238

Fat: 15 g

Carbs: 8 g

Protein: 10 g

Fiber: 4 g

# Spicy Beef Meatballs

Preparation Time: 10 Minutes

Cooking Time: 10 Minutes

Servings: 3

Ingredients:

- 1 cup mozzarella or cheddar cheese; cut into 1x1 cm cubes
- 1 pound minced ground beef
- 1 teaspoon olive oil
- 3 tablespoons parmesan cheese
- 1 teaspoon garlic powder
- 1/2 teaspoon each of pepper, and salt

Direction:

1. Thoroughly combine the ground beef with the entire dry ingredients; mix well.
2. Wrap the cheese cubes into the mince; forming 9 meatballs from the Prepared mixture.
3. Pan-fry the formed meatballs until cooked through, covered (uncover and stirring frequently).

Nutrition:

Calories: 358

Fat: 19 g

Carbs: 4 g

Protein: 18 g

Fiber: 5 g

# Garlic and Thyme Lamb Chops

Preparation Time: 15 minutes

Cooking Time: 10 minutes

Servings: 6

Ingredients:

- 6-4 oz. Lamb chops
- 4 whole garlic cloves
- 2 thyme sprigs
- 1 tsp. Ground thyme
- 3 tbsp. Olive oil

Directions:

1. Warm-up a skillet. Put the olive oil. Rub the chops with the spices.
2. Put the chops in the skillet with the garlic and sprigs of thyme.
3. Sauté within 3 to 4 minutes and serve.

Nutrition:

Net Carbohydrates: 1 g

Protein: 14 g

Total Fats: 21 g

Calories: 252

# Jamaican Jerk Pork

Preparation Time: 15 minutes

Cooking Time: 4 hours

Servings: 12

Ingredients:

- 1 tbsp. Olive oil
- 4 lb. Pork shoulder
- .5 cup Beef Broth
- .25 cup Jamaican Jerk spice blend

Directions:

1. Rub the roast well the oil and the jerk spice blend. Sear the roast on all sides. Put the beef broth.
2. Simmer within four hours on low. Shred and serve.

Nutrition:

Net Carbohydrates: 0 g

Protein: 23 g

Total Fats: 20 g

Calories: 282

# Ketogenic Meatballs

Preparation Time: 15 minutes

Cooking Time: 20 minutes

Servings: 10

Ingredients:

- 1 egg
- .5 cup Grated parmesan
- .5 cup Shredded mozzarella
- 1 lb. Ground beef
- 1 tbsp. garlic

Directions:

1. Warm-up the oven to reach 400. Combine all of the fixings.
2. Shape into meatballs. Bake within 18-20 minutes. Cool and serve.

Nutrition:

Net Carbohydrates: 0.7 g

Protein: 12.2 g

Total Fats: 10.9 g

Calories: 153

# Roasted Leg of Lamb

Preparation Time: 15 minutes

Cooking Time: 1 hour and 30 minutes

Servings: 6

Ingredients:

- .5 cup Reduced-sodium beef broth
- 2 lb. lamb leg
- 6 garlic cloves
- 1 tbsp. rosemary leaves
- 1 tsp. Black pepper

Directions:

1. Warm-up oven temperature to 400 Fahrenheit.
2. Put the lamb in the pan and put the broth and seasonings.
3. Roast 30 minutes and lower the heat to 350° Fahrenheit. Cooking within one hour.
4. Cool and serve.

Nutrition:

Net Carbohydrates: 1 g

Protein: 22 g

Total Fats: 14 g

Calories: 223

# Pulled Pork

Preparation Time: 10 minutes

Cooking Time: 4 hours

Servings: 4

Ingredients:

- 2 lbs. pork shoulder
- 1/3 cup chicken broth
- 1 1/2 teaspoon cocoa powder
- 1/2 teaspoon ground fennel seeds
- 1/2 teaspoon cayenne
- 1 1/2 teaspoons paprika
- 2 teaspoons dried rosemary
- 1 teaspoon garlic powder
- 2 teaspoons onion powder
- 1/4 teaspoon pepper
- 1 tablespoon of sea salt

Directions:

1. In a small bowl, merge together cocoa powder and all spices.
2. Rub spice mixture over pork shoulder. Place pork shoulder in the slow cooked.
3. Pour broth over pork shoulder.
4. Cover slow cooked with lid
5. And Cooking on high for 4 hours.
6. Remove pork from slow cooker and shred using a fork.

7. Serve and enjoy.

Nutrition:

Calories: 679

Fat: 49 g

Net Carbs: 3 g

Protein: 53.8 g

# Mediterranean Lamb Chops

Preparation Time: 25 minutes

Cooking Time: 10 minutes

Servings: 4

Ingredients:

- 8 lamb chops
- 2 tablespoons olive oil
- 2 tablespoons Dijon mustard
- 1 1/2 teaspoon Italian seasoning
- 1 teaspoon garlic, minced
- Pepper
- Salt

Directions:

1. Preheat the oven to 425 F.
2. Season pork chops with pepper and salt and place on a baking tray.
3. In a small bowl, mix together the remaining ingredients and spoon over each pork chops and spread well.
4. Bake for 15 minutes.
5. Serve and enjoy.

Nutrition:

Calories: 391

Fat: 21.2 g

Net Carbs: 1 g

Protein: 48 g

# Oat Bran Molasses Bread

Preparation Time: 10 minutes or less

Cooking Time: 40 minutes

Servings: 8

Ingredients:

- 1/2 cup water, at 80F to 90F
- 11/2 tablespoons melted butter, cooled
- 2 tablespoons blackstrap molasses
- 1/4 teaspoon salt
- 1/8 teaspoon ground nutmeg
- 1/2 cup oat bran
- 11/2 cups whole-wheat bread flour
- 11/8 teaspoons bread machine or instant yeast
- 12 slices / 11/2 pounds
- 3/4 cup water, at 80F to 90F
- 21/4 tablespoons melted butter, cooled
- 3 tablespoons blackstrap molasses
- 1/3 teaspoon salt
- 1/4 teaspoon ground nutmeg
- 3/4 cup oat bran
- 21/4 cups whole-wheat bread flour
- 1 2/3 teaspoons bread machine or instant yeast
- 16 slices / 2 pounds
- 1 cup water, at 80F to 90F
- 3 tablespoons melted butter, cooled

- 1/4 cup blackstrap molasses
- 1/2 teaspoon salt
- 1/4 teaspoon ground nutmeg
- 1 cup oat bran
- 3 cups whole-wheat bread flour
- 21/4 teaspoons bread machine or instant yeast

Directions:

1. Set the ingredients in your bread machine as recommended by the manufacturer.
2. Program the machine for Whole-Wheat/Whole-Grain bread, select light or medium crust, and choose Start.
3. When the loaf is processed, detach the bucket from the machine.
4. Let the loaf cool.
5. Carefully shake the bucket to detach the loaf and set it out onto a rack to cool.
6. Decoration tip: Lightly brush the warm loaf with melted butter when you pop it out of the bucket and scatter toasted whole oats on the top. The butter will create a lovely, soft crust and allow the oats to stick.

Nutrition:

Cal: 137

Total fat: 3g

Saturated fat: 2g

Carbs: 25g

Fiber: 1g

Sodium: 112mg

Protein: 3g

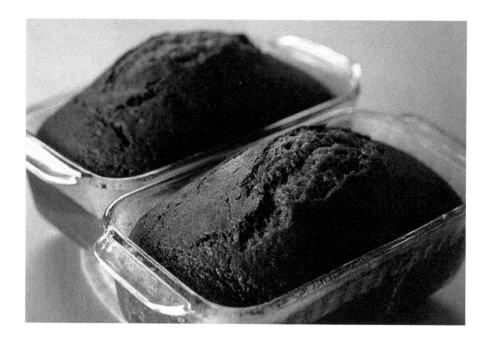

Lightning Source UK Ltd.
Milton Keynes UK
UKHW020802110621
385329UK00001B/130

9 781803 171401